THE WONDERS

OF

GREEN TEA

By Earl Jacobson

Table of Contents

Introduction

Green tea is one of the healthiest beverages, and if we are to rank it – it comes next to drinking water.

By far, it is China and Japan's most drunk tea and has the most significant representation on both China and Japan's most favored top ten teas.

Green tea is proven to be low in caffeine; it also goes through very little processing and oxidization, which means that all the goodness and flavors persevere for you to enjoy in your brew. It is full of antioxidants that have health benefits, which may include:

- Improved brain function

- Fat loss

- Protecting against cancer

- Lowering the risk of heart disease

By reading this book, you will learn about the history of green tea, ten researched health benefits of drinking green tea, types of green tea, and how to brew a perfect cup of tea.

A brief history and overview

The use of tea leaves dates back to southwest China about 3000 years ago. People initially used tea just for chewing and eating; this is similar to how ancient Ethiopians used coffee; they directly ate the coffee beans.

As time went on, the use of leaves and buds started to expand slowly, and people began to use it with other cooking ingredients and added the leaves as flavoring to drinking water.

Methods of green tea preservation can be traced to the 8th century, starting with steaming the leaves to inhibit their oxidation. Later on, in the 12th century, a more contemporary method of firing tea leaves with high heat to kill the enzymes and stop oxidation came into existence.

These two processes resulted in teas that had and still have the characteristic un-oxidized taste. We continue to see both techniques in the production of today's modern teas.

Benefit 1: Contains healthy bioactive compounds.

Apart from helping with hydration, Green tea is a very refreshing beverage. Green tea contains several healthy substances that make it an enjoyable, refreshing beverage. Rich in polyphenols, i.e., naturally existing compounds with health benefits ranging from reducing inflammation to fighting against a range of life-threatening diseases.

Green tea's subtle flavors come from a particular organic compound called epigallocatechin-3-gallate abbreviated as EGCG. Catechins are part of a family of chemicals called flavonoids; they are naturally existing antioxidants that help prevent cell damage and provide other well-documented benefits that give green tea its medicinal properties.

These compounds lead to a reduced formation of free radicals within the body, which increases the protection of cells and molecules from damage. The EGCG in green tea helps treat various diseases; its effectiveness has been researched and well documented.

Green tea also contains small amounts of other minerals such as potassium, calcium, and phosphorous although all of these are in small quantities but can benefit your health.

Given the varied choice of green teas out there, it is essential to note that all teas contain small fluoride amounts. However, there is no need for fluoride levels as it is unlikely to reach levels that would be toxic, but you should be wary of low-grade green teas, though, as they tend to have excessive amounts of fluoride.

In a nutshell, regular intake of green tea has several health benefits due to the concentration of polyphenol antioxidants such as EGCG and several minerals which your body needs.

Benefit 2: Increases fat burning.

If you are looking at the ingredients' list of any fat burning diet, green tea will likely be on that list. According to research, the explanation is quite simple: green tea can increase fat burning and boost your metabolic rate.

In one study involving ten healthy men, taking green tea extract increased the number of calories burned by 4%. In another involving 12 healthy men, green tea extract increased fat oxidation by 17%, compared with those taking a placebo.

However, it is essential to note that some studies on green tea showed no increased metabolism; the effects may depend on the individual. Caffeine may also improve physical performance by mobilizing fatty acids from fat tissue and making them available for use as energy.

Studies have shown that caffeine may increase performance by approximately 11-12%.

In a nutshell, green tea may boost metabolic rate and increase fat burning in the short term; however, remember that not all studies agree with this assessment.

Benefit 3: Improves brain function.

In addition to keeping you alert, green tea does more; it may also help boost your brain function. Caffeine is the essential active compound in green tea; it is a well-known stimulant.

Consumption of caffeine affects brain functions by blocking an inhibitory neurotransmitter called adenosine. Doing so increases the firing of neurons and the concentration of neurotransmitters like dopamine and norepinephrine. Significant research has shown that caffeine can improve various aspects of brain function, such as mood, vigilance, memory, and reaction time.

However, it is essential to note that caffeine is not the only brain-boosting compound in green tea. Another key ingredient in green tea is the amino acid L-theanine, which can prevent damage to cells in the brain by blocking over-stimulation and protecting brain cells from damage due to low oxygen levels. Evidence from electroencephalograph (EEG) studies has shown the existence of a direct effect on the brain. Amounts of the amino acid L-theanine are linked to significant increases in activity within the alpha frequency band, leading to relaxation of the mind without inducing drowsiness.

L-theanine also increases the actions of the inhibitory neurotransmitter GABA and serotonin, which have anti-anxiety effects. In laboratory studies, L-theanine protected cells in the brain region produce dopamine and alpha brain waves.

Several studies show that caffeine and L-theanine can have synergistic effects, which means combining them can have potent effects on improving cognitive function. We now know that green tea may give you a different kind of buzz than coffee because of the L-theanine and small caffeine doses. The majority of green tea drinkers report having more stable energy and being much more productive when drinking tea instead of coffee.

In a nutshell, green tea contains less caffeine than coffee but enough to produce an effect. The amino acid L-theanine in green tea allows it to work synergistically with caffeine to improve brain functions.

Benefit 4: May lower the risk of some cancers.

Cancers are some of the world's leading causes of death. It is a disease or group of diseases caused when cells start to grow uncontrollably, crowding out normal cells. Oxidative damage, i.e., the harm sustained by cells and tissues unable to keep up with the production of free radicals, can lead to chronic inflammation, leading to chronic diseases, including cancers.

Antioxidants can help protect against oxidative damage.
Rich in powerful antioxidants, these substances in green tea inhibit oxidation, especially one used to counteract the deterioration of stored food products.

Research has linked green tea cancer-fighting reputation to the existence of polyphenols, chemicals with antioxidant properties. These chemicals protect the body's cells from free radicals, which are highly reactive molecules responsible for speeding up the damage caused by chemicals in the environment and can lead to cancer development.

Below are some of the studies which have linked green tea to a reduced risk of cancer:

- **Breast cancer**: An extensive observational study review found that women who frequently drank green tea had an approximately 20–30% lower risk of developing breast cancer, the most common cancer in women.

- **Prostate cancer**: One study suggested that green tea antioxidants may prevent prostate cancer growth in men by halting cancer cells' spread and starving the tumor. Recent research shows that the polyphenols in green tea can target the mechanism that triggers cancer spread by stopping the growth of neighboring blood vessels that feed the tumor.

- **Colorectal cancer:** An analysis of 29 studies showed that those drinking green tea were around 42% less likely to develop colorectal cancer.

Green tea needs to be served in its natural form with no additives to achieve the most health benefits. Studies have suggested that the addition of milk to your green tea may reduce its antioxidant value.

Benefit 5: May reduce foul-smelling breath.

Bad breath can be caused by eating or drinking strong-smelling or spicy foods or drinks, gum disease, holes in your teeth, or even an infection. The catechins in green tea have benefits for your oral health.

Studies suggest that catechins can suppress the growth of bacteria, potentially lowering the risk of infections. *Streptococcus mutans*, an oral cavity bacterium, contributes to tooth decay by causing plaque formation.

A cup of green tea contains approximately 200mg of catechins that can inhibit oral bacteria's growth. The efficiency of green tea extract in improving oral hygiene is known for centuries, and this has given researchers that antibacterial activity may be at play.

In a nutshell, the catechins in green tea may inhibit oral bacteria's growth, reducing foul-smelling breath risk.

Benefit 6: May protect the brain from aging.

Apart from improving your brain function in the short term, green tea may also protect your brain as you age.

While the exact cause is unknown, Alzheimer's disease is a neurodegenerative disease and the most common cause of Dementia in older adults. DementiaUK defines Dementia as a range of progressive neurological disorders that affect the brain; these disorders cause brain injuries or diseases that negatively affect memory, thinking, and behavior. There is no cure for Alzheimer's, but green tea is one of the natural remedies that can slow its onset or even the disease's progression.

Parkinson's disease, a common neurodegenerative disease of the central nervous system, is the most common form of Dementia; it involves the death of dopamine-producing neurons in the brain. Smooth and coordinated muscle movements of the body are made possible by a substance called dopamine. In Parkinson's, the cells of the substantia nigra, the part of the brain that produces dopamine, starts to die.

The polyphenols in green tea protect dopamine neurons, and this increases with the amount consumed. These protective effects are associated with the inhibition of the ROS-NO pathway, which may contribute to cell death associated with Parkinson's.

In a nutshell, bioactive compounds in green tea can have various protective effects on the brain. There are reduced risks of dementia-related disorders in older adults who regularly drink green tea.

Benefit 7: May help prevent cardiovascular disease.

Cardiovascular disease can is as a collective term for diseases that affect the heart or blood vessels. Usually, there is an extended build-up of fatty deposits inside the arteries (atherosclerosis), leading to increased blood clots.

Research studies have shown that the catechin compounds in green tea have various protective effects, including lowering LDL cholesterol and triglycerides, which increase the risk of cardiovascular disease.

In a nutshell, bioactive compounds in green tea can have various protective effects on the brain. They may reduce the risk of Dementia and other common neurodegenerative disorders in older adults.

A study conducted on 40,500 Japanese adults concluded that those participants who drank about than five cups or more had a 26% lower risk of death from heart attacks or strokes and up to 16% lower risk of death from all causes compared to people who drank less than one cup a day.

Green tea also raises the blood's antioxidant capacity, protecting the LDL particles from oxidation, one part of the heart disease pathway.

Given the beneficial effect on risk factors, it may not be surprising that people who drink green tea have up to 31% lower risk of dying from cardiovascular disease.

In summary, drinking green tea may improve some of the main risk factors for cardiovascular diseases, including improving total cholesterol and LDL (harmful) cholesterol levels and protecting the LDL particles from oxidation.

Benefit 8: May help prevent type 2 diabetes.

Type 2 diabetes is increasing rate; it causes sugar (glucose) in the blood to become too high. It can lead to symptoms such as excessive thirst, needing to pee a lot, and tiredness. Type 2 diabetes poses an increased risk of getting serious problems with your eyes, heart, and nerves.

Recent studies have found green tea consumption to significantly reduce the fasting glucose and hemoglobin A1c (Hb A1c); overall green tea may improve Insulin sensitivity and lead to a regulation of blood sugar levels.

A study of Japanese individuals found a 42% reduction in the risk of type 2 diabetes in those who drank a lot of green tea.

According to another review of 7 studies with 286,701 individuals, tea drinkers had at least an 18% lower risk of diabetes.

In summary, controlled studies show that green tea may cause mild reductions in blood sugar levels and regulate insulin resistance, leading to a decrease in type 2 diabetes risk.

Benefit 9: May help you live longer.

As we have already seen that some green tea compounds may help protect against cancer and heart disease, it would not be too farfetched to conclude that regular intake of green tea could help you live longer.

If we roll back to the Japanese study mentioned earlier, researchers found that participants who drank a lot of green tea, i.e., five or more cups per day – has a lower mortality rate.

- Death resulting from all causes was 23% lower in women and around 12% lower in men

- Death arising from heart disease: 31% lower in women, 22% lower in men

- Death from strokes: was   42% lower in women, 35% lower in men.

Another study involving 14,001 more senior Japanese individuals found that those who drank a lot of green tea were 76% less likely to die during the 6-year study period.

In summary, the data above show that people who drink green tea may live longer than those who do not.

Benefit 10: May help you lose weight.

Green tea boosts the metabolic rate in the short term. This improvement in metabolism helps those looking to lose weight. It could supplement all other dietary and lifestyle changes you are making to achieve your ideal weight.

Even though studies show modest results, drinking green tea may reduce the build-up of visceral fat, which tends to build around the abdominal area.

A randomized 12-week controlled study involving 240 people with obesity found that those in the green tea group had significantly more decreases in body fat percentage, waist circumference, body weight, and waistline fat than those in the control group.

However, some studies do not show a statistically significant increase in weight loss with green tea, so further researcher needs to be performed in this field to confirm this effect.

In summary, studies show that green tea may lead to increased weight loss. It may exceptionally be effective at reducing dangerous abdominal fat.

Choosing your Green Tea

Deciding which green tea to buy is always a daunting task as there are too many available choices. You would need to choose between loose green tea and green tea bags. While tea bags are more convenient, the loose tea may feel more authentic for a fuller experience of enjoying your green tea. Here are some green tea types you might want to consider:

a) **Dragonwell** – This is a trendy brand of green tea in China. It has a distinctive mellow taste and has a light green flavor. When you add water to this tea, its leaves open to reveal a bud.

b) **Hyson** – This type has a very intense taste and has thick, yellow-green leaves twisted into thin and long shapes.

c) **Gunpowder** – Famously known as "Pearl Tea" in China, this tea resembles tiny gunpowder pellets. The addition of water unfurls the little shells or pearls, and the tea stays freshest longest.

d) **Pi Lo Chun** – This Chinese name translates to "Green Snail Spring." It is a rare fruity tea, and its tiny, rolled leaves look like snails. This tea has fruity flavors of plums, peaches, and apricots embedded in the leaves because the tea bushes for this tea are grown amid orchards.

e) **Matcha** – This tea is in the form of powdered green tea leaves. It appears as a bright green drink.

f) **Gen Mai Cha** – This tea is a combination of sencha tea leaves mixed with fire-roasted rice. It has a savory and earthly taste, and it originates from Japan.

g) **Hojicha** – This is a type of tea with large, unrolled leaves. It has a nutty taste.

h) **Gyokuro** – This is a Japanese green tea with leaves that resemble pine needles; it has a sweet and smooth taste.

i) **Gu Zhang Mao Jian** – This is a unique tea; from silver-tipped young leaves picked within a set 10-day period during spring. Despite being darker than other green teas, it has a smooth and sweet taste.

Brewing your Tea

The brewing process is a simple one as you do not have to worry about common tea additives such as milk, lemon, or sugar, as you should enjoy green tea in its original, pure state.

However, the one thing you might want to account for is how to lessen the amount of caffeine in the pot.

A 230ml cup of green tea contains 8 to 30mg of caffeine. The amount of caffeine present in loose green tea leaves is considerably greater than that present in tea bags. If you find yourself intolerant to caffeine, try reducing your green tea's strength and brew it only on half-strength; of course, you need loose green tea leaves instead of tea bags for this.

Brewing loose tea leaves

Ok back to brewing your tea, it is common for tea drinkers to keep a separate teapot for their green tea to prevent the cross flavoring from black or herbal teas. To get the full flavors from your green tea, be sure to wash your regular teapot well.

You should brew your green tea in ceramic, clay, china, glass, or stainless-steel teapots; avoid plastic or aluminum teapots.

Brewing loose green tea: Add green tea to a tea ball – typically, a spoonful would be adequate. You can drop the tea ball into a teapot for one or two servings if easier but make sure that the capacity for the number of cups you are planning on brewing is adequate.

If you are brewing a single cup, you can drop the tea ball into a cup or mug of freshly boiled water. Be sure to let the water sit for a moment as the ideal brewing temperature for green tea is 82°C (180°F).

Place a lid or plate over the cup except using a tea ball container equipped with a lid or an infuser basket.

Allow your tea to steep for about 3 to 5 minutes except if the instructions state otherwise.
Remove the tea ball and serve.

Brewing green tea bags

Pour boiled water into a cup; let the cup sit for a moment to bring the temperature to about 82°C (180°F)

Now add the green tea bag to the cup of hot water.

Be sure to allow for 3 – 5 minutes for the process of extracting the flavors to occur.

Remove the tea bag and enjoy your drink – some people may also prefer to leave the teabag in the cup.

You should serve green tea usually unsweetened; however, you may add sugar or honey to suit your taste if you prefer.

Conclusion

In conclusion, green tea is a refreshing natural beverage with many benefits such as:

- It is rich in polyphenols to protect against cell damage.

- Has the right balance of caffeine and sustains energy throughout the day without the jitteriness of coffee. Contains EGCG – a master antioxidant, alongside other antioxidants that help scavenge free radicals and have an anti-aging effect.

- It reduces visceral fat, which can aid with weight loss when combined with a nutritious diet and a practical exercise schedule.

- Green ta improves energy and brain function.

- There are various green teas available, but to gain the most benefits, go for high grade-green tea.